The Ultimate Anti-Aging Hacks

The Scientific Approach to Aging Healthier

Jack Benn

TABLE OF CONTENTS

Chapter 1: Decoding Timeless Beauty: Unraveling the Secrets of Youthful Radiance

There is an art in the labyrinth of time where the years leave their permanent markings on our bodies—an art of conserving, enriching, and even rejecting the inevitable aging process. Welcome to the enthralling chapter of "Decoding Timeless Beauty," in which the secrets of young radiance and the science of everlasting charm are revealed.

The Biological Ballet of Aging:

Consider aging to be a delicate dance of biological subtleties, with each movement leaving a mark on the canvas of your skin. Understanding this dance is the first step toward mastering the art of eternal beauty. Collagen and elastin, the dynamic pair responsible for your skin's elasticity and firmness, are at the heart of this ballet. As the years pass, these proteins gradually deteriorate, resulting in wrinkles, drooping, and a lack of youthful bounce.But don't worry; science has provided us with insights into this dance. Researchers have discovered the significance of antioxidants in resisting the damaging dance of free radicals by peering into the tiny realm. These molecular miscreants, which are caused by sun exposure and environmental conditions, lead to accelerated aging. Armed with this knowledge, you can now create an antioxidant-rich skincare program to protect your skin from the tango of time.

The Power of Hydration:

Hydration emerges as a quiet hero in our search for everlasting beauty, soothing the thirst of our skin's deepest layers. Consider your skin to be a rich landscape that wilts and loses its brilliance without adequate hydration. Hyaluronic acid, a naturally occurring component of the skin, acts as a fountain of moisture, absorbing water like a sponge. This reservoir, however, shrinks with age, leaving the skin dry and prone to wrinkles.

Enter the realm of hyaluronic acid-infused skincare, where hydration is elevated to the level of an art form. These compositions, which range from serums to moisturizers, function as moisture magicians, restoring plumpness and suppleness to your skin. Understanding the significance of moisture in ageless beauty entails mastering the chemistry of products that harness its power.

The Collagen Chronicles:

A discussion on everlasting beauty would be incomplete without a look at collagen. Collagen is the structural structure that supports the skin and is sometimes referred to as the "elixir of youth." Unfortunately, the aging story contains a dramatic twist: collagen production declines, resulting in drooping skin and fine wrinkles. But here's the twist: collagen isn't only an outward matter. In this chapter, nutrition takes center stage. Consider your diet to be the screenplay, with collagen-boosting nutrients taking center stage. The foods you eat, from bone broth to omega-3 fatty acid-rich salmon, have an impact on the canvas of your complexion. Furthermore, the market is flooded with collagen supplements that promise a drink from the spring of youth. While these elixirs cannot turn back the clock, they do contribute to the overall story of everlasting beauty. Consider them extras in a big drama of timeless allure.

The Sunlit Symphony:

The sun takes center stage in the play of aging, casting its dazzling beams that, although necessary for life, can also be precursors of skin aging. Consider UV rays to be the antagonists in our beauty story, causing DNA damage, pigmentation, and collagen disintegration. To decipher ageless beauty, you must strike a careful balance between bathing in the sun's warmth and safeguarding your skin from its harsh rays. In this chapter, sunscreen appears as the unsung hero, a vital protector of your skin's youth.

Sunscreen is a ritual in and of itself, a daily commitment to safeguarding the canvas of your beauty. Choose broad-spectrum protection compositions that you can weave into the fabric of your skincare regimen like a favorite thread.

The Rituals of Resilience:

As we uncover the secrets of eternal beauty, resilience rituals take center stage. Consider your skincare regimen a spiritual ritual—a daily commitment to appreciate and safeguard the skin you live in. Cleansing transforms into a cleansing procedure, eliminating the remnants of the day and preparing the canvas for regeneration. The symphony is completed by serums and essences, which give substantial dosages of sustenance and restoration. These formulas are resilience builders, bolstering the skin against the inevitability of time. The night plays out as a pivotal act, with slumber serving as a gateway to regeneration. Consider your skin to be a nighttime garden that thrives in the caring embrace of night creams and treatments.

Beyond the Canvas: Mind-Body Connection:

The mind and body share a delicate dance in the maze of everlasting beauty, shaping the aging story. The silent opponent, stress, writes its narrative on the canvas of your skin. Decoding eternal beauty necessitates not just external cures but also a thoughtful investigation of stress management. Mindfulness practices work like brushstrokes, softening the edges of time. Consider meditation to be a soft caress that smooths away the wrinkles of anxiety and tension. Yoga emerges as a dance, a flowing movement that harmonizes mind and body, encouraging a tranquil demeanor that transcends the rigors of time.

Embracing the Mosaic of Aging:

As we wrap up our look at "Decoding Timeless Beauty," it's critical to accept the mosaic of aging. Each line, each hue, conveys a tale—a story of joy, resilience, and a well-lived life. The search for everlasting beauty is not a mission to erase, but to improve and appreciate the chapters of our lives.

We've unearthed the scientific threads woven into the fabric of eternal allure in this chapter. Each ingredient adds to the harmonic creation of eternal beauty, from the collagen ballet to the hydration symphony, from the sunny story to the resilience rituals. Remember that beauty is a narrative, a story that grows with elegance and

wisdom as you begin on your journey. Decipher the mysteries, accept the rituals, and let your beauty reverberate across the centuries.

Chapter 2: Skincare Alchemy: Beauty from Within

A transformational chapter awaits you in the enchanted realm of skincare, where science meets self-care: "Skincare Alchemy: Beauty from Within."

Consider this a voyage into the alchemical passageways of beauty, where ancient wisdom and cutting-edge technology collide to reveal the secrets of beautiful skin that go far beyond the surface.

The Canvas of Your Skin: A Masterpiece in the Making

Your skin, as a canvas that represents your life narrative, deserves to be embellished with the highest creativity. To begin on this journey toward glowing skin, one must recognize that genuine beauty is more than just skin deep. It's a delicate balancing act between inside energy and outward care—a combination that forms the foundation of skincare alchemy. Let's start with the fundamentals—the pieces that make up this masterpiece. The dynamic combination of collagen and elastin constitutes the structural foundation of your skin. Consider them to be the pillars of a vast mansion. However, as time passes, these pillars tend to sink, resulting in sagging and fine wrinkles. This is where skincare alchemy comes in—a mystical concoction of substances meant to nourish and reinforce.

The Elixir of Youth: Antioxidants and Free-Radical Conundrum

In our search for ageless beauty, we come upon the alchemical marvels of antioxidants—a name that is frequently muttered in the halls of skincare mysticism. These potent molecules fight free radicals, the villainous culprits of accelerated aging, in a heavenly war. Consider free radicals to be renegade components that upset the equilibrium of your skin.

Antioxidants, the virtuous soldiers, neutralize harmful radicals, maintaining the structural integrity of your skin. Vitamins C and E emerge like knights in glittering armor, gracefully brandishing their antioxidant swords. Dive into the alchemical concoctions of vitamin-infused serums and creams, seeing each application as a protective enchantment, protecting your skin from the forces that strive to tarnish its beauty.

Herbal Elixirs and Natural Alchemy

Skincare alchemy dives into the age-old wisdom of herbal remedies—an enthralling combination of nature's richness and ancient traditions. Consider an alchemist's cauldron full of botanical delights such as aloe vera, chamomile, and green tea. Each component not only has a pleasant scent but also a variety of skin-nourishing benefits.

The calming succulent aloe vera is the ointment that soothes sore skin and bestows a cool hug. Chamomile, with its delicate floral scent, is transformed into a potion to soothe inflammation and redness. Green tea, an antioxidant-rich elixir, acts as a protective barrier against environmental stresses. Natural alchemies are the spells woven into your skincare routine that connect you to the ancient whispers of beauty rituals passed down through centuries.

Hydration Magic: From the Depths of the Skin to the Heart of Alchemy

The elixir of life, hydration, lies at the center of skincare alchemy. Consider your skin to be a desert in need of life-giving rain. Hyaluronic acid, a natural component of your skin, acts like a raindrop, infusing moisture into the skin's deepest layers. However, like with any alchemical process, there is a catch: hyaluronic acid depletes with age, leaving your skin thirsty for replenishment. Enter the moisturizing serums, moisturizers, and masks, each drop resembling a fountain of youth. Like experienced alchemists, these compositions seal in moisture, restoring plumpness and suppleness to your skin. Hydration alchemy is more than just superficial dewiness; it's a fundamental communication with your skin's intrinsic capacity to retain and radiate moisture.

Gold Standards and Precious Oils: The Alchemy of Texture

Beyond liquid elixirs, skincare alchemy extends to textures—creamy, velvety, and sumptuous. Consider these textures to be the tactile notes of a symphony, each one essential to the alchemical experience of skincare. Retinoids and peptides, famed alchemical components, build a story of rejuvenation and regeneration. Retinoids, which are produced from vitamin A, appear as alchemists who speed up cellular turnover, revealing younger-looking skin underneath. Peptides, the building components of proteins, act as firmness architects, reducing the appearance of fine wrinkles.

The alchemical brew is enhanced with precious oils produced from seeds and fruits. Consider the opulence of argan oil, the velvety smoothness of rosehip oil, and the golden appeal of jojoba oil.

These oils, which are similar to liquid gold, provide nourishment and luminosity, resulting in a sensory alchemy that transforms your skincare regimen into a self-love ritual.

The Science of Exfoliation: A Ritual of Renewal

Without the ritual of exfoliation—a procedure that parallels the alchemical concept of transformation—skincare alchemy is incomplete. Consider exfoliation to be an alchemist's elixir that reveals the radiant layers beneath, removing the dull and worn surface. Alpha and beta hydroxy acids (AHAs and BHAs) act as alchemical agents, dissolving dead skin cells and unveiling the brilliance concealed inside. AHAs, such as glycolic and lactic acids, dance on the skin's surface, providing a mild exfoliation that boosts brightness. BHAs, like salicylic acid, penetrate your pores, purifying and refining them. This alchemical exfoliation dance is a transforming act, a ritual that revitalizes weary skin and prepares it for the absorption of future skincare enchantments.

From Alchemy to Ritual: Crafting Your Skincare Symphony

As we wind our way through "Skincare Alchemy: Beauty from Within," it becomes clear that this journey goes beyond the humdrum application of creams and serums. Skincare alchemy is a ritual—a symphony of textures, fragrances, and sensations that elevates your self-care regimen to the level of an art form. Consider your skincare regimen to be a personal alchemy laboratory, with each product representing a vial of strong elixirs ready to be combined. The art is not just in the application but also in the attention that goes into each step.

As you cleanse, imagine not just your skin but also your spirit being cleansed. Feel the alchemical process taking place at the cellular level when you apply serums. As a result, the canvas of your skin becomes a work of art—an alchemical creation that reflects the balance of inner life and exterior care. In the realm of skincare alchemy, beauty is a journey, an ongoing investigation of the ever-changing

relationship between you and your skin. May
each potion and ritual you create as you begin on
this alchemical journey be a celebration of the
dazzling, timeless beauty that lives inside.

Chapter 3: Nutrition for Ageless Living

One consistent thread threads through every chapter of life's kaleidoscope: the desire for everlasting vitality. As we progress through our lives, the importance of nutrition becomes more apparent. This chapter takes us on a trip into the heart of ageless life via the lens of nourishment—a voyage that transcends traditional temporal bounds and embraces the essence of holistic well-being.

The Symphony of Nutrients

To comprehend everlasting existence, we must first decipher the symphony of nutrients that our bodies require. Consider nutrition to be the conductor of a musical dance of vitamins, minerals, antioxidants, and macronutrients. Each note is critical to preserving the balance of our physiological and psychological well-being.

Mindful Eating: A Ritual of Reverence

In today's fast-paced world, eating has become more of a chore than a ritual. However, in the pursuit of eternal living, the act of feeding oneself becomes a holy ritual—a celebration of life itself. The cornerstone of this practice is mindful eating, which encourages us to relish every meal and fosters a connection between our bodies and the nourishment they receive. Consider a dish full of vivid veggies, nutritious grains, and lean proteins—a canvas painted with the colors of longevity. It's not just about the food on your plate; it's about adopting a

way of life that recognizes the body's requirements and the journey toward everlasting vitality.

The Fountain of Youth in Every Bite

Our nutritional choices have enormous power, serving as an elixir that feeds the spring of youth inside. Berries high in antioxidants, omega-3 fatty acids found in fatty fish, and a colorful

variety of vegetables are not just ingredients;
they are the keys to unlocking the body's
potential for an ageless existence.

Consider the avocado, a creamy miracle that not
only thrills the tongue but also provides
necessary fatty acids to the skin. Or the simple
sweet potato, which is high in beta-carotene, a
precursor to the skin-beneficial vitamin A. These
culinary treasures are more than simply a treat
for the taste senses; they are a bargain with time,
promising to infuse our bodies and brains with
youth that knows no age.

The Dance of Gut Health and Longevity

The stomach takes center stage in the delicate
ballet of ageless existence. The microbiome, a
teeming community of billions of bacteria living
in our digestive tract, is more than just a
biological sidekick; it is a pivotal figure in the
story of lifespan.

The things we eat influence this microbial
metropolis, affecting everything from

immunological function to mental health. Fermented foods, with their probiotic brilliance, emerge as the microbial heroes of this story. Yogurt, kimchi, and sauerkraut aren't just tasty treats; they're also anti-inflammatory buddies and gut-balance keepers. We fuel our bodies while simultaneously cultivating a vibrant ecosystem within, one that reflects the vitality we want in the fabric of ageless life.

Hydration: The Elixir of Eternal Youth

The elixir of perpetual youth, in the search for timeless life, is a simple yet strong elixir—water. Hydration is the hidden hero of anti-aging life—a liquid ally that lubricates joints, feeds the skin, and energizes every cell. It's not just about drinking enough water; it's about nourishing our bodies with the life-giving essence of pure hydration. We enable our bodies to perform properly by sipping from the cup of renewal. Water is more than simply a drink; it is a lifeline that transcends age, reminding us that the cornerstone of ageless existence resides in nature's simplest and purest components.

Navigating the Culinary Landscape: A Tapestry of Flavor and Health

The gastronomic scene is broad, full of options that may either accelerate us to an ageless life or lead us astray. It's a tapestry woven with strands of flavor and health, and our decisions define the masterpiece of our well-being. Consider the Mediterranean diet, which is composed of olive oil, fresh fruits and vegetables, and lean meats. This culinary marvel is a global beacon of age-defying sustenance, not simply a localized treat. The Japanese embrace the longevity-promoting properties of shellfish and fermented soy, creating a gastronomic culture that whispers the secrets of eternal youth.Let us remember, as we navigate this culinary maze, that each meal is an opportunity—a chance to nourish our bodies with nutrients that transcend time, an opportunity to leave a legacy of ageless life through the artistry of our choices.

The Alchemy of Adaptogens

Adaptogens appear as the alchemists in the everlasting living narrative, refining the essence of resilience and vigor. These botanical miracles, ranging from ashwagandha to rhodiola, are more than just supplements; they are the keepers of balance in the face of life's turbulent currents. As stress, a constant foe, strives to undermine our well-being, adaptogens serve as staunch defenders, bolstering our bodies and brains against the ravages of time. Consider drinking a cup of tulsi tea, the leaves of which whisper stories of ancient wisdom and perseverance. Consider the power of ginseng, a natural ally that has been passed down through centuries, delivering the gift of vigor and adaptability. We uncover a potent elixir in the alchemy of adaptogens that allows us to handle the ebb and flow of life with grace and ease.

The Tapestry of Ageless Living

Each dietary decision, thoughtful bite, and nutrition ritual adds to a legacy that transcends time in the magnificent fabric of ageless existence. It's a tapestry made with threads of vivid veggies, omega-3-rich fish, fermented foods' probiotic dance, and hydration elixir.

Our dietary choices are brushstrokes on this canvas, portraying an image of energy that transcends age stereotypes. Let us remember, as we dig into the complexities of nutrition for ageless living, that this is not simply a chapter in the book of life—it is the tale itself. It's a tribute to the body's tenacity, a hymn to the ageless energy that lives within. So, let us taste each meal, enjoy the nutritional symphony, and dance with the adaptogens, for in the kaleidoscope of ageless life, we discover the real artistry of sustaining the body, mind, and soul across the pages of time.

CHAPTER 4: Mind-Body Harmony: Stress, Sleep, and Beyond

The delicate tango between mind and body frequently falters in the fast-paced rhythm of modern living. Stress, like a looming shadow, disrupts the peaceful harmony that should exist between our mental and physical environments. This chapter takes us on a trip through the intricate tapestry of mind-body harmony, navigating the tumultuous waterways of stress, exploring the lands of restoring sleep, and transcending into the infinite vistas beyond.

The Symphony of Stress: A Modern Malady

Stress, an ever-present companion in modern life, is more than simply a psychological burden; it is also a physiological disruptor. In its never-ending quest for productivity, the mind mistakenly activates the body's stress response, triggering a chain reaction of hormonal and neurological reactions.

Consider the body to be a beautifully tuned instrument, and stress to be the discordant note that disrupts the entire symphony. The adrenal glands, like conductors, emit a flood of cortisol and adrenaline to prepare the body for a perceived threat. This stress reaction is adaptive in the short term, a survival strategy encoded in our DNA. In the chronic tempo of modern existence, however, it becomes a malady, a constant drumming that resonates throughout our everyday lives.

Cultivating Calm: The Art of Stress Management

To restore balance in the mind-body symphony, we must become calm artisans, wielding instruments that dispel the stress storm. In this creative attempt, mindfulness meditation, an old technique now accepted by contemporary science, appears as a powerful brushstroke. By focusing our attention on the present moment, we may quiet the clamor of worried thoughts and restore the mind to its natural state of balance. Consider the maze of lavender fields, their aroma drifting into the air—a time-tested natural treatment. Lavender essential oil harnesses the magic of aromatherapy, urging us to inhale calm and exhale stress. These simple yet profound activities become threads in the tapestry of stress management, weaving a fabric of tranquility in the face of life's obstacles.

Sleep: The Restorative Symphony of the Night

Sleep, as the night's restorative symphony, takes center stage in the vast composition of mind-body harmony. In the stormy sea of modernity, however, restful sleep frequently eludes us, leaving our minds and bodies trapped on the beaches of exhaustion. The significance of sleep goes beyond ordinary rest—it is a trip our bodies do each night, a holy trek into the regions of regeneration. During the peaceful hours of the night, the body engages in a dance of repair and restoration. Cells rejuvenate, memories solidify, and the mind spins a tapestry of dreams. It is not simply a halt in the symphony of life; it is the crescendo that assures the music continues. As we go deeper into the realms of sleep hygiene, we come across the need for a constant sleep schedule—a rhythmic cadence that synchronizes our internal clock with the cosmic pulse of night and day. The faint illumination of electronic displays creates a disruptive dissonance in this nocturnal symphony; hence, disconnecting before bedtime develops as a holy rite, helping the mind to effortlessly shift from the rush of the day to the peace of the night.

Beyond Sleep: The Horizons of Holistic Well-being

Mind-body harmony involves the complete well-being of the person and goes beyond stress management and decent sleep. Physical exertion becomes a joyful dance in this broad setting, an expression of energy that surpasses the confines of ordinary exercise. Movement becomes a celebration of the body's power for joyful expression, whether in the shape of a brisk stroll, the fluidity of yoga, or the beat of dance. Consider the ancient martial technique of tai chi, which resembles a slow, contemplative dance. Tai Chi's careful motions harmonize the breath, body, and mind, providing a route to balance and centeredness. It is more than just a workout; it is a moving meditation that invites us to embrace the wholeness of our being.

The Nutrition-Mind Connection: Fueling the Mind-Body Symphony

The threads of mind-body harmony weave through the nutrition fabric because what we eat is more than just food—it is the fuel that fuels the mind-body symphony. Omega-3 fatty acids, which are prevalent in fatty foods such as salmon and walnuts, serve as lyrical notes that boost cognitive function and emotional well-being. The delicate ballet of mood regulation is formed by the complicated dance of neurotransmitters, which is dependent on a consistent supply of amino acids from protein-rich foods. Antioxidants emerge as the protectors of brain health in the big feast of life, shielding the sensitive neurons from the oxidative stress that life's difficulties bring. The bright spectrum of fruits and vegetables, with their rich phytonutrient palette, becomes a painter's brush, creating a work of cognitive vigor art.

The Mind-Body Connection: A Tapestry of Resilience

The connection between mental and physical well-being appears as the golden thread in the weaving of mind-body harmony—a thread that, when fostered, generates resilience and energy. Instead of being a strong antagonist, stress serves as a teacher, helping us toward attentive reactions and adaptive coping techniques. Sleep, rather than being a biological requirement, becomes a divine rite that heals the soul. Let us remember, while we negotiate the maze of contemporary living, that the symphony of mind-body harmony is not a faraway melody—it is the very heartbeat of our existence. It is an invitation to embrace the ebb and flow of life's trials and delights by dancing to the beat of life. We discover an eternal harmony in the union of mind and body that transcends the confines of time, reverberating through the corridors of our being as the melody of everlasting life.

CHAPTER 5: Revolutionizing Fitness for Age-Defiance

In the grand scheme of things, the search for age defiance is an eternal voyage that invites us to push the limits of what's possible. As a steadfast partner on this journey, fitness transcends the usual bounds of sweat and repetition—it becomes the spearhead in the revolt against time constraints. In this chapter, we begin on a transforming journey into the domain of age-defying fitness, exploring the human body's untapped potential and rewriting the script of what it means to age.

The Evolution of Fitness: Beyond Muscles and Mass

In the history of fitness, the emphasis was frequently on chiseled muscles and Herculean strength. While the visual attractiveness of a well-defined body remains, the paradigm of age-defying fitness encompasses resilience, flexibility, and functional strength. It's a movement that calls into question the idea that aging must imply decline—a call to arms to recover the energy that is properly ours. Consider fitness not as a punishing chore, but as a freeing force—an ally who enables us to move through life with grace and enthusiasm. The revolution begins with a shift of perspective: moving from seeing exercise as a chore to seeing it as a celebration of what the human body is capable of.

Functional Fitness: Navigating Life with Grace

Functional fitness emerges as the North Star in the quest for age defiance—a strategy that teaches the body to excel in daily tasks. It's not about bench-pressing enormous weights, but about being able to move groceries, mount stairs, and turn with agility. It's a revolution that takes fitness out of the gym and into the huge arena of real-world functioning. Consider the simplicity of bodyweight workouts, in which the body provides the resistance. Push-ups, squats, and planks serve as the fundamental bricks in the functional fitness castle, promoting strength that extends beyond the bounds of individual muscles. We rediscover the joy of movement in this revolution, appreciating the body's intrinsic capacity to negotiate the complexities of daily living with grace.

The Art of Flexibility: Bending, Not Breaking

Aging does not have to be linked with stiffness; it may instead be a journey into the art of flexibility. Yoga takes center stage, urging us to extend beyond our imagined constraints and embrace the suppleness that resists the passage of time. Yoga is more than just a physical exercise; it is a comprehensive journey that combines breath, movement, and awareness. Consider the warrior position, which not only strengthens the legs but also builds mental fortitude. The slow flow of sun salutations becomes a dance with the morning, pouring vigor and peace into the body and spirit. Yoga becomes the weaver in the tapestry of age-defying fitness, weaving flexibility into the very fabric of our being—a tribute to the body's ability to adapt and flourish.

*Resilience Training: The Mental Fortitude
Revolution*

The anti-aging revolution is not limited to the physical domain; it also includes mental fortitude. The capacity to recover from life's challenges, or resilience, becomes the hidden weapon in the armory of age-defying fitness. Much like a muscle, the mind may be taught to weather storms gracefully and emerge stronger on the other side.Consider mindfulness meditation to be a revolutionary practice that rewires the neural pathways of the brain, not a passing fad. We create an anchor in the silence of meditation that roots us in the present moment, allowing us to confront problems with a calm and cool attitude. It's a revolution that goes beyond the cacophony of stress, cultivating mental fortitude that becomes a cornerstone in the building of age-defiance.

Innovative Modalities: The Technological Frontier

The age-defying fitness revolution extends into the technology frontier, where innovation becomes a catalyst for transformation. Virtual reality exercises, activity monitors, and tailored training applications are reshaping the fitness scene, allowing for a more dynamic and adaptable approach to fitness. The conventional gym is no longer the sole realm of age-defying warriors; the revolution is now available to everyone, whether at home or in the enormous expanse of virtual places. Consider the gamification of exercise, in which training is transformed into a fun experience rather than a tedious habit. Virtual reality simulations take us to realms where physical capabilities are pushed to their limits and the search for health is linked with the excitement of discovery. Technology becomes a facilitator in this transition, moving us toward age-defying innovation and drive.

Nutrition as Fuel: The Powerhouse of Age-Defiance

Nutrition emerges as a powerhouse in the global anti-aging revolution—a crucial force that drives the body's resilience and vigor. It is more than just counting calories; it is about adopting a dietary philosophy that nourishes the body from the inside. Fruits high in antioxidants, lean proteins, and a diverse range of vegetables serve as artillery in the fight against oxidative stress, a strong opponent that hastens the aging process. Consider the Mediterranean diet not as a restricted diet but as a new way of life that combines flavor with health.

With its monounsaturated fats, olive oil transforms into an elixir that nourishes the skin and promotes cardiovascular health. In moderation, red wine becomes a toast to the longevity revolution, with its polyphenols forming a protective barrier against the ravages of time.

Community and Connection: The Social Revolution

The anti-aging movement extends beyond the person to the social fabric, where community and connection serve as catalysts for age-defying vitality. Group exercise programs, community sports leagues, and shared health journeys all contribute to a supportive environment that encourages people toward age-defying objectives. Consider the impact of friendship in a cycling class, where the group enthusiasm acts as a propellant for each individual. The social revolution in fitness is about establishing connections that inspire, encourage, and lastly, not just share sweat sessions. The threads of community become the brilliant hues that fill the path with pleasure and resilience in the fabric of age-defying fitness.

The Age-Defying Mindset: A Revolutionary Paradigm Shift

The ultimate revolution in the broad tapestry of age-defiance is a paradigm shift—a shift in attitude that rejects the concept of aging as a decline. It's a drastic break from cultural narratives that depict aging as a sunset; instead, it's a celebration of the sunrise, a declaration that the finest chapters are yet to come. Consider George Bernard Shaw's words: "We don't stop playing because we grow old; we grow old because we stop playing." The age-defying attitude is a movement that sees life as an ever-changing adventure, a chance to explore, learn, and reinvent what is possible. It's a proclamation that fitness is a journey, not a goal, one that changes, adapts, and transcends temporal constraints.

The Age-Defiance Revolution

In the big story of age-defying, exercise appears not as a mere tool but as the revolutionary force propelling us to the pinnacle of life. It's a trip that goes beyond the traditional limits of physical capability and gets into the whole essence of well-being. The anti-aging revolution is a collaborative effort in which each note, stride, and mentality adjustment contributes to the harmonic harmony of age-defying existence. Let us embrace the revolutionary energy that is inside us as we embark on this transforming journey. Let fitness be the banner we wave in the face of aging, a declaration that we are designers of our fate, sculptors of our vitality, and revolutionaries in the vast story of age-defiance.

The path is not without hurdles, but with each stride, each revolutionary workout, and each shared moment of triumph, we go closer to a horizon where the bounds of age are but a mirage in the sands of time. "The Ultimate Anti-Aging Hacks" explores the intriguing realm of defying time and discovering the keys to living a youthful and vibrant life. This book, written with an intelligent perspective on holistic well-being, provides a thorough guide to not only appearing younger but also feeling younger from the inside out. In the first few chapters, the author lays the groundwork by delving into the science of aging. They examine the biological mechanisms, free radicals, and hereditary variables that contribute to the aging process using simple terminology. What distinguishes this book is its dedication to bridging the gap between scientific study and practical application, making it a great resource for readers from a variety of backgrounds.

Beyond the technical language, the book easily turns into practical tactics. The author calls for a comprehensive strategy that considers physical health, mental health, and lifestyle choices. Each chapter is a treasure trove of concrete information, ranging from food suggestions based on anti-inflammatory principles to mindfulness activities that encourage stress reduction.

"The Ultimate Anti-Aging Hacks" explores cutting-edge technology and treatments, which is one of the book's main characteristics. The author goes into new skincare trends, hormone therapy, and tailored medicine. The book helps readers make educated judgments about adopting these advances into their personal anti-aging path by demystifying these advancements. Throughout the story, the author provides anecdotes and success stories, which lend a human touch that readers appreciate. These real-life examples not only inspire but also give context for the book's techniques. The conversational tone of the writing fosters a bond between the author and the reader, making the anti-aging journey feel like a shared experience. The book navigates the subtleties of fitness and exercise in the context of aging as it proceeds. The need for personalized fitness programs that adapt to individual requirements and tastes is emphasized by the author. From strength training to yoga, the book calls for a more diverse approach to physical activity that goes beyond traditional exercise stereotypes.

With entire chapters devoted to cognitive exercises, mindfulness techniques, and sleep management, the comprehensive approach also addresses mental wellness. By discussing the relationship between the body and the mind, the author supports the notion that real anti-aging entails fostering resilience in both the body and the mind. Another noteworthy aspect of "The Ultimate Anti-Aging Hacks" is its dedication to diversity. The author acknowledges that anti-aging tactics ought to be appropriate for a wide range of users. Regardless of the reader's age, the book offers personalized guidance that considers the reader's particular situation and objectives. Practical recommendations, such as building individualized anti-aging programs and making tiny adjustments gradually, elevate this book from a theoretical investigation to practical guidance. The author recognizes that the route to aging gracefully is not one-size-fits-all and urges readers to embrace their individuality. The book's concluding chapters examine cultural attitudes toward aging and dispute the prejudices that frequently accompany growing older. By encouraging a positive and empowered attitude toward aging, the author invites readers to redefine their relationship with time and embrace each stage of life as an opportunity for growth and fulfillment.

"The Ultimate Anti-Aging Hacks" concludes with a resounding call to action, urging readers to embark on their anti-aging journey with confidence and curiosity. The author's voice, a blend of expertise and genuine enthusiasm, permeates every page, making this book not only an informative read but also an uplifting and empowering one.In essence, "The Ultimate Anti-Aging Hacks" transcends the typical boundaries of self-help literature. It is a holistic manual that empowers readers to take charge of their aging process, armed with knowledge, practical strategies, and a newfound sense of confidence. Written with a captivating blend of scientific rigor and relatable anecdotes, this book is a timeless guide for anyone seeking to defy the conventional constraints of time and embrace a life of vitality and well-being.